THE DOCTOR AND
THE SOCIAL SERVICES

UNIVERSITY OF LONDON
HEATH CLARK LECTURES 1969
delivered at
The London School of Hygiene and Tropical Medicine

The Doctor and the Social Services

by

R. HUWS JONES

National Institute for Social Work Training

UNIVERSITY OF LONDON
THE ATHLONE PRESS
1971

Published by
THE ATHLONE PRESS
UNIVERSITY OF LONDON
at 2 Gower Street, London WC1

Distributed by Tiptree Book Services Ltd
Tiptree, Essex

Australia and New Zealand
Melbourne University Press

U.S.A.
Oxford University Press Inc
New York

© *University of London* 1971

ISBN 0 485 26322 X

Printed in Great Britain by
WESTERN PRINTING SERVICES LTD
BRISTOL

CONTENTS

CHAPTER I

I. INTRODUCTION: THE TIMELINESS OF THE TOPIC

THE THEME of the Heath Clark Lectures for 1969 is collaboration between the health services and the other social services. At present, each group has only a meagre and patchy knowledge of what the others can provide. With some splendid exceptions, even when they know each other's resources, they rarely use them. There is mutual suspicion where there should be co-operation and as a result, the community fails to achieve the health or welfare that it might. Patients and clients suffer more and longer than they need.

One task for us all in the next few years is to create the conditions for more effective teamwork than we have today. This will in part be a matter of structure, organization, and management. But it also involves, for all concerned, basic questions about professional attitudes and about the purpose that our services exist to promote in our affluent, complex, and torn society. It involves questions about professional education and re-education and how to monitor innovation and design operational experiments that will enable us to substitute evidence for assertion.

My theme is not a new one; much has been written about it by some who are in this audience, including my Chairman.[1] Unlike the pavement artist, I should display a notice saying 'Emphatically not all my own work'. I would indeed be daunted but for the fact that no one can deny that we need to look at this theme again, and this should be a propitious moment.

For forty amazing years medical science and arts have concerned themselves with chemo-therapy and with dazzling developments in surgery. No one who has listened to surgeons

[1] Professor J. N. Morris, Department of Public Health, University of London and Director of the Social Medicine Unit of the Medical Research Council.

and medical scientists who are working with tissue transplantation talk about the significance of renal transplantation for the mother with a young family can doubt their passionate concern with the personal and social significance of their work. Nevertheless, compared with medical advances in the first quarter of this century, the tide of interest and endeavour has been away from social aspects. Today there are clear signs that this interest is renewing—as it must, if the effects of 'scientific' medicine and surgery are not to be lost. Ferguson and others [1] have provided disturbing evidence that what the hospital can achieve in therapy, the careless community can destroy again in a few months through poor after-care or none at all.

This is a good moment for looking again at the relation of health to the other social services partly because almost every family doctor you talk to tells you that his main jobs today and for the foreseeable future lie not so much in coping with dramatic episodes and people who are acutely ill but with long term patients, people handicapped in body or mind, the aged infirm who will live on for a decade or more. It is helping people to live with situations—not just diseases—which will continue as part of their lives and helping to prevent these situations from deteriorating; this task calls for a team that includes a variety of fellow workers. Society, it has been said, [2] is moving towards a symbiosis which sees the physician, the teacher and the social worker as social service professionals with common objectives; some would wish to see the architect, the planner, the priest, and the administrator within this symbiosis.

Because health and social welfare share a common interest and commitment, it does not follow that all social problems are primarily medical. All problems affecting the welfare of human beings have a physical aspect and also economic, legal, ethical, and social aspects and an aspect that some would call spiritual. No one aspect has the right to claim an absolute, invariable, or infallible priority of concern—though all in turn have done just this.

My subject is 'The Doctor and the Social Services', and of course medicine has always been part of the community's social provision. Karl de Schweinitz [3] tells how a Statute of 1414 called for a reform of hospitals which, said the preamble, were established '. . . to sustain impotent men and women, lazars, men out of their wits and poor women with child, and to nourish, relieve and refresh other poor people'. Hospitals, as the origin of the word indicates, were first founded to provide a home for poor and homeless people; medical attention was added later. Poverty, indeed, was the great illness though affluence has not proved to be the great cure. The close connection between health and welfare is original and built-in and, if denied, it re-asserts itself irresistibly, even in the U.S.A. where a recent official report [4] says that 'medical care is becoming an increasingly important part of social welfare.'

2. DOCTORS ARE SCARCE AND DEMANDS AND EXPECTATIONS ARE GROWING

We are experiencing an escalating demand for medical services. For a great number of years the demand for doctors will increase more than proportionately to their numbers in Britain and in those richer countries that compete for British doctors. The recent U.S. report 'Services for people' [4] lists the trends affecting the social services and puts first the 'increasing demands by the population for health services'; another trend is the declining ratio of physicians to all other health personnel, the ratio in the U.S.A. being already one to ten.

The increasing demand for the services of doctors is apparently not due to the spread of the malady known as hypochondria. Professor Butterfield [5] is one of the latest to draw attention to the serious failure of people with complaints to use appropriate medical agencies; from his enquiry it appears that only about half of those with complaints were being treated, and only 16 per cent with medicines prescribed by doctors. We have all heard of the icebergs of hidden disease; each new epidemiological survey identifies more. Brotherston [6] says that a major phenomenon of the elderly is their under-demand of the national health services.

Twenty years ago Aneurin Bevan commented that the National Health Service had made suffering articulate. Ignorance, however, has proved a powerful inhibitor, though it may now be declining: consultation rates for ill-defined

conditions tend to be higher among the young and middle
aged than among the elderly; and young adults in the less
skilled occupational groups, having known the National Health
Service for as long as they can remember, seem readier to
consult a doctor than their parents were [7].

The future promises a scarcity of doctors, increasing readiness
to use them—whether appropriately or not—and rising expectations of what doctors can do, especially in the area we euphe-
mistically describe as 'mental health'. Cartwright [8] found that
some 40 per cent of patients thought a general practitioner a
suitable person to consult about their difficult children or their
difficult spouses. And doctors themselves are increasingly aware
that inevitably they are intervening in social situations for which
they are not altogether equipped. The point was made recently
by R. D. Laing [9] who wrote:

When a doctor, in a purely medical capacity, diagnoses tonsillitis in
a child, or cancer in an adult, and orders them-into hospital for
investigation and operation, he is clearly intervening in a social
situation to which, however, he usually has neither the time, nor the
interest, to give more than passing notice . . . 'purely' medical
decisions have massive reverberations in a whole network of people,
with consequences to many others than the patient alone . . . social
reverberations . . . are, more often than not, left to reverberate away.

A well placed medical observer told me of increasing satisfaction among family doctors when their work is so organized that
the practice operates as a team with other professional people:
the practice nurse, the district nurse, the health visitor and the
social worker. But the picture of increasing demand and rising
expectations to which I have referred must be seen against the
more general background of dissatisfaction in family practice.
This, it is suggested, is related in part to the fact that family
doctors spend only one-sixth or less of their time doing medicine
as they have learnt it [5]. One consultant psychiatrist, appointed
medical superintendent to a hospital, said he spends at least as
much time on jobs like marriage guidance and in the administration of what is really hostel accommodation in disguise. Here
is frustration, potential damage, and waste. Medical practitioners, always too few and hard pressed, use their training in
only a small part of their professional practice and spend much

time on work for which they are neither trained nor think they should be trained.

Obviously, the inappropriate use of medical time exaggerates the scarcity of doctors. A high proportion of medical men in family practice and hospitals fail to recognize the extent to which their partners—or potential partners—in other professions could do some of the things that they are trying to do and do some of them better.

3. THE DOCTOR'S KNOWLEDGE AND USE OF THE SOCIAL SERVICES

General practitioners and hospital consultants seriously fail to call on social services that their patients need even when they are there to be used. Rodgers and Dixon [10] surveying services in a small county borough in Lancashire, said that the most striking fact was 'the sketchiness of the doctors' knowledge of the social services'. Jefferys [11] said of Buckinghamshire, that enterprising county, that many doctors confessed ignorance of the services and how they could be mobilized on behalf of their patients. Meyrick and Cox [12] wrote in the *Lancet* in 1969 of 'colossal ignorance' in the London Borough of Lewisham about services available from local authorities—and they did not exempt the general practitioners.

Ferguson [1] and his colleagues reported that one quarter of patients discharged from hospital deteriorated seriously within three months, and they suggested that relapse is due as much to poor home conditions and failure of after-care as to any inevitable progress of the pathological condition. Hard evidence comes from the work of Anderson and Elizabeth Warren [13] recently of the Public Health Department of this School. They listed eleven community services, every one of them linked closely with health, such as home helps, meals-on-wheels and chiropody. Of the family doctors who responded to the enquiry, only about one-third had full working knowledge of more than seven of these eleven services and one-third had working knowledge of only five or fewer. With a flair for understatement, the authors comment that 'If the family doctor is to play a significant part in making health and welfare services available to patients who require them, then he has to know where to apply for help.' They go on to say that the replies indicated that many doctors were positively reluctant to suggest appropriate services and that this reluctance indicates that they were not oriented towards these services.

The implications are serious: people who are sick and vulnerable are not being helped to get services even when they are available for them and scarce medical resources are not being used as they should be. Evidence has been accumulating—by now it ought to overwhelm us—about large numbers of hospital patients who are old, chronically ill and physically or mentally handicapped, for whom further active medical treatment is unlikely to produce results. As their needs are no longer primarily medical, life outside the hospital—and this would often be possible given support from the social services—could mean a livelier life, it might be less expensive and would to some extent free hospital beds for people who need treatment that can be given only in hospital.

4. EXAMPLES

As a result of medical and social improvements, the care that is needed today, especially from family doctors, is typically long-term care and this can bring severe strain for families and communities. Examples flock so hard that the difficulty is in selection.

A decade ago, few children with spina bifida survived beyond the first two months; today, because of early surgical intervention, two-thirds survive at least five years and increasing numbers live to adolescence and longer [14, 15]. Spina bifida is proportionally more common in industrial areas in the western half of the country such as South Wales; the risk of a second spina bifida birth is relatively high, about 1 in 15.

Here is a medico-social problem with profound ethical and policy implications, as recent correspondence in the *Lancet* has shown [16]. A high proportion of spina bifida children are paralysed, deformed in the legs and incontinent; at present about one-third are retarded mentally. Most of these children live at home and few family doctors, or even local hospitals, have the experience and knowledge to help parents adequately with the strictly medical problems, quite apart from the emotional, economic and social strains. The studies in South Wales by Hare, Laurence and their colleagues, with which I have had the privilege of being associated, show clearly the need for the co-ordinated provision of medical and social help to the whole family: birth control advice is needed, including genetic counselling; the family's expenses are high, partly because of recurrent hospital visits; the physical strains will be heavy; the parents will have lasting anxieties about the attitudes of neighbours and school authorities and later about employment; there are disturbing effects on marital relations and on the other children and there is the recurrent and agonizing question 'would it have been better if we had said no to the operation?'.

Social services are available to help with many—though not all—of these needs; new services, such as the mutual comfort that can come through a parents' association can be created; but the study in South Wales shows that parents are *not* adequately advised and often the varied forms of help that they and the patient need are not called upon even when they are available.

Paraplegia provides another example. At one time, patients with traumatic paraplegia were likely to die within a year of injury. Thanks to medical progress, a much higher proportion now survive, three-quarters live at home and two-thirds are gainfully employed. Outside specialist hospitals, few have close knowledge and experience of this condition yet the management of paraplegia in the community depends on the careful and sustained teamwork of the patients and those responsible for them: the family doctor and the district nurse; housing departments; local authority departments which provide special equipment, occupational therapists, home helps, social casework for the social and psychological problems of adjustment for patients and relatives; the retraining and employment services and social security officers. A recent article by Forder and his colleagues [17] shows that even with the impetus that comes from a specialist paraplegic centre, a total of only four contacts were made with the local authority services by the eight general practitioners involved in this enquiry.

It may be said that spina bifida and paraplegia are rare conditions though the problems they illustrate are increasingly common. Old age, however, is a risk we all run today, for during this century we have as a community enabled some four grandparents to grow where only one grew before. Here all the problems meet, for 'old age never comes alone' and disabilities which people cope with when they are younger, advance with age until they become oppressive and perhaps unbearable.

Family doctors see old people more than any other workers in the public services, more even than the officers of the Supplementary Benefits Commission. They could be a key element for linking with essential social services, especially for vulnerable groups such as those leaving hopsital or living alone in advanced old age. However, recent work by Brocklehurst and Shergold [18, 19] showed that 37 per cent of old people discharged from hospital did not see their general practitioner within the first month after discharge and a writer in *The Practitioner* [20] said that these especially vulnerable groups among old people may in practice come to the attention of a local authority welfare officer rather than their family doctor.

A study of services for old people has just been completed by the National Institute for Social Work Training in co-operation with the London Borough of Southwark and with support from the Department of Health and Social Security [21]. It was found that only one-third of the old people who applied to the welfare department for assistance were referred by health agencies of any kind and most of these referrals came from hospitals. Although one half of the sample were already receiving at least one domiciliary service, in almost every case there was need for more services, many of which were actually available in the borough. The Director of the project and the medical member of the team were impressed by the attitude of hopelessness towards old age which was common among the family doctors who, it was thought by the doctor in our team, assumed too readily that in view of the patient's age and infirmity it was not worthwhile to try a hearing aid, arrange for a functional assessment or refer a depressed old person to a psychiatrist for therapy.

The workers in the project comment on the 'comforting

assumption' that you can do nothing until your old patients come to you. On the other hand, in those cases where family doctors, hospitals and domiciliary health and welfare services were able to collaborate, the results were rewarding in promoting specialist medical treatment and social support. The study also shows that, for their part, the social workers were not quick enough to appreciate the medical needs of old people and help them to go for examination and treatment. This research, which is now being written up, confirms the impression that more aggressive medical and social action is needed, not to prevent old age, for we know only one way of doing that, but to prevent, reduce or compensate for some of the disabling accompaniments of old age.

One of the hardest moments even in a long life comes when old people recognize that they can no longer go on living independently. Perhaps they could manage if they had more domiciliary assistance—a home help, meals-on-wheels, a home nurse, a health visitor, calls from a voluntary worker, more neighbourly support, transport to a club, etc. Or is it better for them to move to live with a relative, remembering that the pattern traditionally preferred by those who *can* choose is the dower house, near to but not part of the younger family? Should they go into what we rather oddly call 'sheltered housing' or should they enter residential accommodation, which for them has the considerable disadvantage that it is full of old people? Or is some other alternative more suitable, such as boarding with a host family, a private hotel or nursing home or a home for the mentally frail? These are desperate decisions, even for those who have loving and knowledgeable friends to help them decide.

The starting point, though this is often ignored, ought surely to be a medical assessment which, in many cases, should include a psychiatric examination. But Kay, Beamish and Roth [22] have pointed out that 'there is unfortunately very little contact between psychiatrists and geriatricians, although both are concerned with large numbers of patients suffering from quite similar disorders'.

A full social assessment also should be taken for granted and there ought to be one person, able to act as a member of the

team, who knows the range of services and who has the understanding and skill necessary to help the old man or woman sort
out the realistic alternatives, help them to *try* some if they want
to, ensuring if humanly possible that a genuine choice is open
to them. This same person should also be responsible for seeing
that the agreed solution is carried out or should know the
reason why, for decisions may be left in the air; they should
ensure that plans are reviewed from time to time and rarely
should any decision be treated as final.

5. DOCTORS ARE IN A GOOD POSITION TO MAKE OTHER SERVICES KNOWN

Doctors are in a unique position to promote the use of services.
To begin with, 98 per cent of the population is registered with
family doctors. Moreover, it has been said [23] 'An outstanding
feature of the values that prevail in our society is the respect-
ability of ill-health . . . association as patients with doctors is a
thing to boast about.'

Today we are, I hope, moving away from the old principle
of less eligibility, designed to discourage people from using the
social services, to a new principle of more eligibility, making the
services readily available and encouraging those who need them
to use them. This new approach means that we should attach
personal social services to acceptable points in the social system
such as general practice, where it was found in one recent
enquiry that 70 per cent of patients referred to a social worker
were not in touch with any of the other social services [24].
Titmuss has suggested that the more the family doctor gets
mixed up in community care, the more chance he has of helping
to set standards for other professional workers [2] and, we may
add, contributing through their prestige towards improving
their local services where they are poor or insufficient.

6. SOCIAL WORK AND ITS CONTRIBUTION

I have—almost gingerly—kept away from the term social work.
This is not by accident. My theme is the connection of the
doctor with the other personal social services and with some

that, curiously enough, are regarded as less personal, such as housing and income maintenance. If this connection is to be effective it must, of course, engage the doctor's lively interest in the services as they reach his own patients; it also implies a continuing contribution to the current debates through which old policies for these services are re-examined and new ones hammered out, at local as well as national level.

Many workers are involved in these services: for instance, the staffs of day centres, including play centres and day nurseries; home helps and their organizers; administrators and receptionists, and all kinds of workers in the field of residential care. However, the position of the social worker is central and signal. Their functions—and what are not their functions—are not always understood, especially perhaps by their admirers. English history records an official called the Keeper of the King's Conscience. It must have been a hot seat! Today there is a tendency to make social workers the keepers of society's conscience—or to regard them as a kind of social tranquillizer. In debates in Parliament it is alarming to hear it taken for granted that stubborn social problems would melt away if only we had more social workers to reform the nuisances and the threatening characters, but leaving the rest of us comfortably as we are. Perhaps equally dangerous is the assumption that because it is sometimes a social worker's role to try to reconcile the demands of society and of deviant individuals and groups, social work is, therefore, primarily an agent of social control.

On the other hand, social workers are not simply disposal officers, clearer-ups of hospital beds nor are they there simply to lay on practical help just as they are told to.

What positively can the social worker contribute towards the care of the doctors' patients in general practice, in hospital, and in community medicine? The Younghusband Report [25] comments that the young general practitioner may at first be overwhelmed by the magnitude of the social problems arising in his practice. This danger, I suggest, is not confined to general practice, the young practitioner, or 'at first'. The skilled social worker can help in assessing the patient's social situation and— given the time—can estimate its material and personal strength and weakness, the relationships within the family, the work situation, the influence of neighbourhood and social class, the patient's and the family's liability to stress.

It is the business of the social worker (though there are indications that this has not always received the attention it merits) [26] to know the available range of appropriate services—statutory, voluntary and organized good neighbourliness—and how to mobilize them; this is no easy task today when the services are complex and even baffling. Ideally, and here I try to set out the ideal, the social worker should be alert to important needs for which there are no adequate services and should seek ways of filling the gaps, in individual cases and—working with colleagues—through changes in provision and policy. It is, however, not enough to set out the services available to the patient and his family. Help from the doctor and the social worker may be wanted, even by well informed and intelligent people, in the painful business of reviewing their own situation and deciding between the appropriate and acceptable alternatives. A patient who is very disturbed may not be able to make rational use of the resources that are there to assist him; the social worker may then need to help the patient to express his anxieties and untangle his wants. As in all professions, social work carries an ombudsman function; it should ensure that the client knows his rights, if necessary it should encourage him to exercise them and make sure that they are provided if they are wanted. There is also the obligation to review the situation and check the effectiveness of the plan of action or at least make sure that the patient knows how to get in touch if need be. It has been said [27] that social workers should evaluate and make known what social services do *to* people in doing things *for* them.

It is perhaps the core of social work that it aims to increase people's understanding of themselves in relation to their own situation and to other people and to help them when these relationships are disturbed.

The goal of social work then is to assist people, in co-operation with medical and other services, with social and personal aspects of their problems which they cannot solve without help. Some of these problems are created and many are exacerbated by other contemporary social changes: by geographic and economic mobility; by our galloping technology; by the doctor's ability to help people survive who not long ago would have died; by our determination to create environments—in high flats or concrete communities, without knowing what they do to those who live in them.

7. SUMMARY

In response to sustained expressions of the will of the people, Parliament has this century evolved a comprehensive national health service and a range of other services, incomparably better than any previous generation has known. The achievements of these services are not acknowledged as often as their weaknesses, but they are so great that, for instance by extending life, they contribute substantially to our current problems. These achievements leave us puzzled and sometimes indignant about our failures—about revelations like Ely [28] (which was not so much revealed as *seen*, at last) and the fact to which our Chairman has drawn attention in the *Lancet* [29], that the number of old and elderly people in hospitals for the mentally ill and handicapped has risen sharply over the last five years.

One obstacle which prevents the country from reaping a full return from its investment in the health and welfare services is the inability of different workers to understand the contribution that others could make to their work, and the consequent failure to mesh these services together reliably for the benefit of the patient.

I have referred to several studies that draw attention to this weakness and have tried to show that a team approach is indispensable by examples which, though rare in themselves, illustrate a much wider group. I have also tried to illustrate by referring to very old people who, in number and probably in the severity of their need, constitute the dominant group for the health and welfare services—a group that is here to stay and which will grow in number for as long as will interest most of us, at least professionally.

Doctors, I have urged, are in a unique position to make other social services known to those patients who need them; the doctor's prestige could contribute impressively towards improving the services in those areas where they are poor.

What factors account for this weakness in co-operation and what action—or even thought—could help? These are questions for the next two chapters, but a brief 'trailer' may be indicated.

We should dismiss the idea that indifferent collaboration can be explained in terms of anybody's fault. Here is but one example of the general problem of relations between professions, indeed of departmentalism in modern society, a problem that is likely to baffle us for many a day.

Some elements are simple to set out if not to cope with. The present pattern of the social services makes them notoriously hard to know and to use. Difficulties of communication, within professions as well as between them, are now receiving attention, especially in the hospital service. At least one study shows that mistaken impressions and unreal expectations about what other workers do are today a powerful impediment to useful communication.

Social services are not likely to be used consistently if the doctor finds them slow to respond, inflexible, unaccommodating or unreliable. The community social services have been starved of resources, especially for the training of their staff, and this must be remedied. In proportion to its population, one local authority recently spent only one-twenty-fifth as much as another authority on its home help service; authorities at the bottom of this kind of league-table can be very bad indeed.

But even in the best endowed areas, there are not and there never can be enough resources to match all needs; cost benefit analyses or some comparable methods must be devised to guide political and professional judgment on how resources can best be used to meet need and, since these services *must* be rationed, the rationale of the rationing must be understood by those who apply it and it must be made clear to other people.

Differences between professions can be powerfully affected by the assumption, which I shall want to challenge, that basic differences yawn between them in their ethical codes and practice.

Unlike social workers, doctors as a profession have a very long history and, especially in the last hundred years, have acquired immense prestige and authority. From this derives the assumption, referred to in a *Times* leader [30], that doctors have an automatic right to the captaincy of any team to which they belong. The whole concept of 'captain' in this context may need to be examined.

Improved collaboration should come through more rational structures for the services, through clearer communication and by working out—by recorded experience as well as by operational studies—the criteria for recognizing those cases where teamwork is necessary. The active involvement of workers from different services in debates on policy and planning at all levels would contribute greatly.

But as a shoemaker, I must affirm that there is nothing like leather: we shall know each other's services better and use them more effectively for the advantage of our patients and clients when learning about these other services is recognized as an indispensable element in our professional education. It will not be easy to carry this out with the required economy of time and effort and every teacher of professional practice knows that classroom teaching and reading, though essential, are not enough. Students may be taught—and they may pass examinations—and yet find themselves clueless in applying what they have learnt. The skilful teaching of inter-professional practice, I shall suggest, calls for a new type of centre for the study of such questions as, what are the characteristics of those teams that do work together successfully, how can fresh experiments be promoted at the grass root level, and how can we learn quickly from them; how can the *continuing practice* of teamwork be taught, not only in education that leads to professional qualifications but in the successive re-tooling operations now seen to be necessary in all professions. This new centre for interdisciplinary practice might contribute to a fresh concept, the idea of *families* of professions, instead of the strictly individualistic and compartmentalized concept of professions that we have at present.

Finally, I shall wish to look at new patterns of collaboration that are now emerging or that might emerge through new structures, new forms of organization and other influences, patterns that will we hope make for more fruitful partnership between social services and doctors, whether they are based in family practices, in hospital or in community medicine.

REFERENCES

1   FERGUSON, T. and McPHAIL, A. N. (1954) *Hospital and the Community*, London: Oxford University Press.
2   TITMUSS, R. M. (1968) *Commitment to Welfare*, London: George Allen & Unwin.
3   DE SCHWEINITZ, K. (1943) *England's Road to Social Security*, University of Pennsylvania Press.
4   TASK FORCE ON SOCIAL SERVICES (1968) *Services for People*, U.S. Dept. of Health Education and Welfare.
5   BUTTERFIELD, W. J. H. (1968) *Priorities in Medicine*, London: Nuffield Provincial Hospital Trust.
6   BROTHERSTON, J. H. F. (1969) 'Change and the National Health Service', *Scottish Medical Journal* **14**, 130.
7   OFFICE OF HEALTH ECONOMICS (1963) *The Personal Health Services*, London: Office of Health Economics.
8   CARTWRIGHT, A. (1967) *Patients and their Doctors*, London: Routledge and Kegan Paul.
9   LAING, R. D. (1969) *Intervention in Social Situations*, Association of Family Caseworkers.
10 RODGERS, B. and DIXON, J. (1960) *Portrait of Social Work*, London: Oxford University Press.
11 JEFFERYS, M. (1965) *An Anatomy of Social Welfare Services*, London: Michael Joseph.
12 MEYRICK, R. U. and COX, A. (1969) 'A Geriatric Survey Repeated', *Lancet* 7 June 1969.
13 WARREN E. A. and ANDERSON, J. A. D. (1966 & 1967) 'Communications with General Practitioners', *The Medical Officer* 16 Dec. 1966 and 21 July 1967.
14 LAURENCE, K. M. (1967) 'The Central Nervous System Malformations and their Family Problems', *Mother and Child* **39**.
15 HARE, E. H. and LAURENCE, K. M. (1969) 'The Parents of the Child with Spina Bifida Cystica', *Paediatric Digest* Feb.
16 *The Lancet* (1969) Letters to the Editor on Spina Bifida.
17 FORDER, A. *et al.* (1969) *Communication in the Health Service*, Social and Economic Administration vol. 3 no. 1.
18 BROCKLEHURST, J. C. and SHERGOLD, M. (1968) 'What Happens when Geriatric Patients Leave Hospital?', *Lancet* 23 November.
19 BROCKLEHURST, J. C. and SHERGOLD, M. (1969) 'Old People Leaving Hospital', *Gerontologia Clinica*.
20 MORTON, E. V. B. and BARKER, M. E. (1968) 'The Present Nonsense and the Elderly Sick', *The Practitioner* vol. 200.
21 GOLDBERG, E. M. *et al.* (1970) *Helping the Aged: A Field Experiment in Social Work*, London: George Allen & Unwin; National Institute for Social Work Training Series.

22 KAY, BEAMISH and ROTH (1962) 'Medical and Social Character-
    istics of Elderly People under State Care', Keele University: *The
    Sociological Review* no. 5.
23 WILSON, R. (1963) *Difficult Housing Estates*, London: Tavistock
    Pamphlet no. 5.
24 GOLDBERG, E. M., *et al.* (1968) 'Social Work in General Practice',
    Lancet 7 September.
25 *Report of the Working Party on Social Workers in the Local Authority Health
    and Welfare Services* (1959) H.M.S.O.
26 MOON, M. (1964) *The First Two Years: A study of the work experience
    of newly qualified medical social workers*, London: The Institute of
    Medical Social Workers.
27 TOWLE, C. and PERLMAN, H. H. (1969) *Helping*, University of
    Chicago Press.
28 *Report of Committee of Enquiry into Allegations at the Ely Hospital, Cardiff*
    (1969) H.M.S.O. Cmnd. 3975.
29 MORRIS, J. N. (1969) 'Tomorrow's Community Physician', *Lancet*
    18 October.
30 *The Times* Leader, 4 July 1969.

CHAPTER II

I. OBSTACLES TO CO-OPERATION: WEAKNESSES IN THE SOCIAL SERVICES

TEAMWORK between the health and social services ought to be the regular practice whenever it is required for the benefit of patients or clients. This opening sentence would be banal as well as tautological except that what should be the rule is in fact rare. Of course, there are the conspicuous exceptions; Marjorie Warren's pioneer work with old people, in which she established the custom of frequent and genuinely co-operative sessions with social workers and through them with other social services; the tradition of inter-professional collaboration founded by Spence in work with young children and their families in Newcastle; examples of effective teamwork in child guidance, in a few group general practices and in some imaginative joint endeavours in community mental health.

This failure to establish a regular pattern of working together should not be attributed simply to the perversity of social workers or doctors, though doubtless both have their share of that characteristic; human nature is very prevalent, even in the professions. There are more important influences than other people's cussedness, their determination to build empires or preserve them, more significant factors than personal immiscibility or professional jealousies; we shall be groping for explanations for a long time.

A host of reasons, connected with communication, professional codes and attitudes, organization and training can be advanced to account for failure in co-operation, and some of these will be considered shortly. But, in spite of deeper and more subtle explanations for the indifferent use of services, I believe there'd be a revolution in their use *if* . . .; if they were simple to know and easy to get at; if they were dependably there, sufficient to meet real need and reasonably sure to respond quickly, and if doctors and their patients were convinced that these services produced results.

Good wine needs no bush but even thirsty people may not return if the wine is off, or the cask empty. The personal social services are so organized—if that is the right word—that it is hard for anyone to see them as a rational structure; they are difficult to understand and doctors (like other people) complain that the appropriate services are hard to find. One group of family doctors was asked 'Would you use the services more if there was just one number to dial?' The answer came quickly 'It would never stop ringing!' And the answer conveys warning as well as promise for social services are complex to use and only for the simple situation is there a simple solution.

The community services have been starved of resources— especially for training staff, and this is the more significant in services like these where, to a large extent, the staff is the service.

How far are the services today equipped to respond when, for instance, the doctor asks for a home help? Independent estimates indicate that over the country as a whole we require about twice the number of home helps to meet the clear needs, so that a lot of people who should have home helps do not get them. Not long ago, one town in England spent £480 per 1000 of the population on home helps; another, similar in size and social composition, spent £17, less than one-twenty-fifth as much. Part of the justification of local government is that it does permit wide differences between authorities, but differences of this order, and they are not confined to home helps, raise urgent questions about whether the minimum should be tolerated.

More resources for the social services are essential but there may never be enough to respond to all the demands and better services create more demand [1]. When it is not possible to meet needs, doctors—and the direct consumers—should be told *why*. Rationing is unavoidable; if it is not planned and explained it is much more likely to be and seen to be arbitrary and unfair. This comment is all the more relevant now we know that local authority social service departments are to be established; if the history of the National Health Service is anything to go by, the increase in the demand for services will be significant and it could prove overwhelming.

It is also said, and with justice, that social workers are not to be found where the need for them is greatest. Like people in other professions they prefer to live in the more agreeable parts of the country; and Tizard [2] for instance, has pointed out that the provision of social casework for the families of severely retarded people, always inadequate, is if anything worse now than it was ten years ago. It has been suggested that what is happening is that, because of the increase in the number of severely retarded people who live longer, a growing amount of social casework has had to be shared amongst a much more rapidly growing number of people needing help. Some of these grounds of complaint should disappear when the structure of the social services is no longer based on superficial symptoms or other arbitrary classifications of people in need.

It takes a lot to provoke the ordinary human being to the point of recording a complaint and I doubt if criticisms of the social services, whether by doctors, other professionals or the public, are generally treated with the high seriousness that complaints ought to receive, especially where the consumer lacks the ultimate control of taking his business to another concern. In some of the more efficient ventures in big business, I have been told, they have devised ways of reaching out to find complaints and dissatisfactions even before the consumers have formulated them, and then responding to what they find. For many years operative statistics have been used in big business, for instance, and by some university public health departments to make comparisons between organizations and within organizations. These operative statistics are designed not just to show how good an establishment is but especially to disclose its weakness to itself, to point up plainly where it is least effective, where it fails to match changing demands. This use of operative statistics has begun in the personal social services, and inevitably begun through somewhat general academic studies; but very few if any local authority social service departments have started to use this method as a regular means of testing their own performance.

Here is an attempt to grab initiative by the forelock: not to leave it to blow like the wind where it listeth but to plan for initiative, to build it into the organization. But it is necessary to add a warning. There is a kind of Gresham's law at work 'daily routine drives out planning'. If we are to have vigorous built-in initiative in our social welfare services there should be units whose first responsibility is to review activities, make comparisons, anticipate needs, look where growth is wanted and—no less necessary—consider regularly which services can now be cut back or done away with.

2. COMMUNICATION

It was, I think, a character in the *New Yorker* who complained that the worst thing about people who can't communicate is that they never stop talking; we may sometimes feel the same about institutions. In any case the comment serves to remind us that the problems of communications are even more complex than most people assume. Important studies have been carried out in the health service, and especially in hospitals, about how communication works (and fails to work) at present and how it can be improved—between staff and patients, staff and staff, and between the hospital and the outside world. [3]

The consultants in the paraplegic centre to which I referred earlier [4] saw the family doctor as having an overall responsibility for bringing in skilled personnel from other services and they took for granted a co-ordinating function which, in practice, was accepted by only one general practitioner out of eight. Other impediments to good communication which that study showed had not received attention were the very large area covered by this centre, crossing the perils of several administrative boundaries, and the sheer complexity of the management of paraplegia in the community. These factors could be peculiar to the work of this centre but one suspects they have wider implications.

Difficulties of communication can arise between, for example, medical and social workers, even on the goals and methods which they presume they have in common. To quote an example given by Hooper [5], the social worker may wish to increase the independence of a patient, supposedly in the interests of recovery, whereas the doctor and nurse may well wish to diminish this, again in the interest of recovery. Good communication may lead to understanding that *both* types of approach are acceptable at different points in time in the treatment regimen.

Brevity (as every lecturer should remind himself) is the soul of consideration and doctors in all branches have complained that when they consult social workers the reports they receive, verbal and written, are inordinately long and show little consideration for the size and pressure of the doctor's workload.

In short, this is a plea for more studies, outside the hospital system as well as within, of problems of communication between members of the helping services and those they serve, remembering that ineffective communication with *patients* and their relatives, still a recurring criticism, is likely also to impede communication between doctors and the other services. Examples include the oddly hostile reception accorded to the Central Health Services Council's report on communication between doctors, nurses and patients [6] and the same reaction occurred to the earlier production of the short document on *Human Relations in Midwifery* [7] by the Advisory Committee on Maternity and Midwifery.

3. ORGANIZATION AND POLICY

Godber [8] has said that '. . . individuals will only get what they need in this complicated world of medical service if competent, understanding men have organized the deployment of mutually supporting services to that end'. Organization, of course, is essential and it can never be neutral; organization influences the quality of relationship between all concerned. The present organization of the health services has been damned most authoritatively in the Green Paper [9] and the organization of the personal social services in the Seebohm Report [10]. Organizations which ought to encourage adaptability, in practice preserve a static situation, resistant to change from without and within. But these problems are by no means confined to health and social services or to the United Kingdom. Official committees of enquiry similar in scope to the Seebohm Committee, are found today in several European countries, in the U.S.A. and in Commonwealth countries.

Complaint comes first about the plethora of separate services, about complexity and the lack of clarity of purpose and provision as these services present themselves to the public and to workers in other fields. In one sense these services *have* to be complex if they are to be geared to their task but, like the television or the motor car, they do not have to be that complicated to use.

Today there are administrative, financial and professional pressures which discourage authorities from taking decisions solely because they are best for the patient, family or community. The classic example, used *ad nauseam* but one that must be used until it is no longer relevant, refers to infirm old people. One famous hospital has complained that it has 15 to 20 beds always occupied, for an average of 14 months, by old people who do not need hospital care. On the other hand, welfare authorities complain of difficulties in getting old people into hospital though they need nursing that the Home cannot provide. It was in this context that years ago the *Manchester Guardian* coined its famous leader headline: Death by Administrative Failure. This administrative blockage has been there long enough to justify surgery.

In general, the danger is that the administrative and financial framework, without which there can be no service, may distort the substance of the service itself and impede co-operation. And perhaps there can be no final answer to this except 'eternal vigilance'.

For twenty years we have had what Kenneth Robinson [11] once described as interdependent but separately managed streams of care. What matters to the patient or client and his family is how far these streams flow together in practice and to a great extent this determines the returns the country gets from its investment in the services.

The situation is illustrated in provision for mentally handicapped people where the streams of care have remained very separate. The contemporary review begins, nearly forty years after the courageous report of the Wood Committee on Mental Deficiency [12], with the epidemiological material which Kushlick and his colleagues [13] are now providing. How many retarded people do we have, and with what degrees of severity? How are they distributed, geographically and by income or occupational groups? What are the trends and how are they likely to be affected by internal migration, by preventive factors which seem to have been successful in the last thirty years [2] in reducing the proportion of babies born with severe mental handicap and on the other hand those factors which favour the survival of defective children who would otherwise have succumbed, especially to respiratory diseases. Then comes the hard question about where does it seem best for severely retarded children and adults to live, for their own sake and for the sake of their families and what would they choose if choice were available? The answer—which can rarely be simple or confident —obviously depends on what support is provided in the community, how good—or how horrifying—the institutional care seems to be and how easy it is for the patient in the community to re-enter hospital or hostel at short notice if the circumstances of the family make this necessary. This question, especially if we think about it in relation to people we know personally, forces us to consider whether any human beings should pass their lives in hospitals or in any institutions that seem like hospitals, unless they require active treatment that cannot properly be provided outside.

Medical men and laymen are now asking what precisely is the specialist role of the doctor or nurse in the residential care of mentally handicapped people of any age, beyond the stage of initial assessment and the periodic checks on the progress of any physical disability. Of course, like everyone else, mentally handicapped people need their family doctor and district nurse, and will need consultants from time to time.

Reports such as the one on Ely Hospital and Pauline Morris's book *Put Away* [14, 15] force us to ask whether tolerable conditions can possibly be assured for staff if we have agglomerations of several hundreds of these inevitably difficult patients on one site; above all the staff must be helped to retain their interest, their patience, their resilience and sheer physical efficiency. The active involvement of the families of the patients, the neighbourhood and local industry must be engaged, both because of what it brings positively into the lives of the patients and for the safeguards it introduces in case things go wrong. Ely, said the Report, was a closely knit and inward looking community, lacking the participation of other statutory and voluntary services.

This illustration, topical and perhaps already too familiar, shows that we can't have quite separate and still sensible policies for severely retarded people, one for hospitals and one for local authorities. We need the contributions of different services provided as parts of a co-ordinated plan and this will not emerge as a result of instant alterations in existing provision introduced to meet demands stimulated for instance by scandals in the Sunday newspapers.

The mutual involvement of doctors and other social services in the field of policy could do much to determine whether the 'totality of care' becomes a reality; we need effective teamwork for planning, no less than for the care of the individual patient.

The term policy, of course, should not be confined to major discussions of government, professional organizations or local authority councils. Every general practice, hospital department, voluntary organization and local social service department, has a policy, even if it is only the determination never to recognize it or admit it. Doctors, working with the other social services, could do much to identify the unmet needs in particular areas. By their professional competence and by their prestige they could contribute to develop the more adequate, comprehensive and co-ordinated services which they, more than most people, know to be necessary.

It is by the struggle to define and analyse these policy questions in a dialogue between the professions, administrators, politicians and the public, that we shall be helped to decisions, eventually we hope based on evidence of effectiveness, about where the priorities for new allocations and reallocations of resources should go: to hospitals or to housing? how much to health education and how much to medical training? more into higher sickness benefits, into family practice or into industrial medicine? more into geriatric beds or into domiciliary services? more into residential accommodation or for social work staff? These are some of the questions the relevant professions must study together if we are to achieve an integrated policy and not just respond erratically to day-to-day pressures.

4. PROFESSIONAL PRIDE AND PREJUDICE

Looking for reasons for poor collaboration between doctors and workers in other services, we have reviewed certain weaknesses in the social services, and some impediments in communication; we have also looked at the influence of organizational structure and the way policy is made at various levels. Two factors of exceptional importance remain, one is the complex of professional influences; the other and closely related factor is professional education.

The difficulty of co-operation between doctors and workers in other social services is just one illustration of the wider problem of co-operation between professions and even within professions, a problem that will grow if, as Carr Saunders [16] prophesied, professions must multiply in the sort of society we are creating. Professions are, in fact, a dangerous necessity. It was Shaw in *The Doctor's Dilemma* who said that all professions are conspiracies against the laity; and all can become associations for spreading the doctrine of self importance. Professionalism, with its characteristic suspicion and hostility to other professions, is related closely to the malaise of departmentalism, one of the most insidious influences in our managerial society.

Some of the incompatibility between medical and social work springs, of course, from the relative ages of the two professions. Each in its turn has struggled out of an era of do-it-yourself, or get in a neighbour who has the knack. But this struggle dates back more than two millenia for medicine and barely a hundred years for social work.

We think, perhaps naïvely, that common aims should prove a powerful link; in fact, common knowledge and skill, even the common use of a vocabulary which one profession regards as its patent, may be an impediment, putting professions in apparent competition, as can be read in the history of relations between doctors and midwives or the more recent uncertainties in the relations between health visitors and social workers.

If we start with the assumption that wide differences exist between professions in their code of ethics, this also will prove a barrier to co-operation; worse still, it may be used to justify a refusal to co-operate. It can be argued that the ethical basis of all professions is and must be essentially the same. The ethical problem is always a choice between alternatives, as illustrated by a medical friend who said that for him the touchstone was, are you only for the patient? 'If I'm satisfied you are', he said, 'then I'm likely to share confidential information; if not I won't share it, even if you are a doctor.' This is part of the dilemma: are we likely to help the patient best if we look at the problem only from his point of view, ignoring his family, his school or work-place and his neighbourhood when the trouble is for example mental ill health or venereal disease? The answer cannot be easy.

Here I should like to quote Brotherston who wrote [17]

What about the traditional one-to-one responsibility of medical practice? According to this the doctor is responsible for his individual patient and for him only. Actually, of course, the profession's definition and responsibility has never been quite as narrow as that. It has always accepted some degree of community responsibility, for example, in the control of infection. How does the interpretation of responsibility run in a community health service? The profession must cling to its Hippocratic tradition to do its utmost to help each patient. But at the same time there is plenty of evidence in the Health Service, that in so doing we may be doing less than our best for people in the queue who have not yet become our patients (Felstein, 1964).

The views of the Seebohm Committee on confidentiality, one aspect of professional ethics, have been much misunderstood— or misrepresented. The report acknowledges the tradition which leads to the present difficulties, but argues that it derives from views of professional practice that are increasingly anachronistic. Today, problems of any seriousness are rarely dealt with by individuals but by *teams* and confidential information is exchanged freely, otherwise the work could not be done properly. The current conflict derives in part from real or assumed differences in professional status and these will not disappear until social workers, doctors, teachers, nurses, administrators and others realize that they are all members of a team and accept the team approach to family problems. 'A new code of practice is essential', says the Report, 'to meet the changing situation and we think the professions concerned should initiate discussions among themselves, and with members of the public through which such a code could be formulated.'

This year the *British Medical Journal* [18] reported a discussion in the General Medical Services Committee of the B.M.A. in which P. M. Crawford said:

that 'Social workers were much more concerned about the problem of confidentiality than doctors were, and their standards of confidentiality were even higher than those of the medical profession. He had found sometimes that that worked to the detriment of the patient, because he had been without information which would have been of value.'

Other members of the Committee spoke on similar lines.

Samuel Johnson once described patriotism as the last refuge of the scoundrel; he might think again if he could hear the letter of professional ethics used in *all* professions to oppose the spirit of collaboration. But, thank goodness, professional practice is often much better than precept and one exceptionally informed social worker tells me that in her experience the issue of confidentiality has in fact never once arisen where social workers and doctors work closely together.

In an ideal world professions should develop, as part of their ethic, a built in self-criticizing mechanism. In practice, professional bodies do not conspicuously work that way and none but the boldest administrators fulfil this role in public. It is therefore arguable that what we need increasingly is more inter-professional criticism as a 'quality control'. The development of inter-professional criticism, as well as collaboration, is one safeguard against unbalanced administrative and political interference. It is also a safeguard against legalizing consumer complaint to the point of hostility. Even more important, is the way in which the acceptance of inter-professional standards could lead to more effective quality controls in professional behaviour generally.[1]

Who is to be leader in any health and welfare team is a delicate and difficult question which I would dodge altogether if I dared. But the issue crops up all over the place, from Todd

---

[1] I am indebted to R. M. Titmuss for suggesting points in this paragraph.

to *The Times* and the issue is too important to be left to resolve itself for, says Brotherston [17]

> If the team is small enough and close enough, decisions may come automatically from like-mindedness. But when the team becomes large, heterogeneous and scattered . . . effective decision making may be hampered, and reduced to neutral compromise. The medical profession . . . cannot afford to postpone the development of devices of leadership which can give full effect to interdependent teamwork.

I shall return to this issue later.

Meanwhile, may I recall that the Todd Report [19] tackled this question as early as paragraph 29, saying: 'A separate but related development is the increasing need for the doctor to work in close co-operation, both in diagnosis and in therapy, with people who are not medically qualified—not only with the scientists whose contribution to clinical assessment is becoming increasingly important, but also with the many others who have important responsibilities for the patient both in ancillary services and in other capacities, and above all with the patient himself.' Later the Report says, in one of the most quoted passages, 'The leadership that the doctor often has to exercise has sometimes in the past appeared to be based on the assumption of a charismatic authority which has already ceased to be convincing and in the future will be completely inappropriate.'

Issues like this are affected quite a bit by the precise words we use, and terms like 'supplementary professions' and 'ancillaries' are not helpful. Social workers are accused of being unreasonably touchy when they express their fears of becoming 'handmaidens' in a situation in which they have their own unique contribution to make, and not simply one that doctors or other workers could make if only they had the time. It must be recognized that in different circumstances the major contribution may come from different professions. Titmuss [20] has suggested that we need a careful and authoritative enquiry to define and clarify the many different components of responsibility. 'Such an enquiry would have to take account of responsibilities which relate, first, to the *ascertainment and diagnosis* of social and medical need, secondly, to the *initiation* of action to see that needs are met, and thirdly, to *continuity* of action to see that effective and co-ordinated use is made of the services available.'

In his training, the doctor today is taught to ask for evidence, to distinguish between unverified assertion and theories which have been tested by systematic observation and experiment. He asks—or the layman hopes he asks—just what difference does this make, and what about the side effects? Experimental science, said Roger Bacon in the thirteenth century, alone gives certainty to the conclusions which other sciences reach by argument. But it was only 100 years ago that medical scientists reached a stage which would be regarded as experimental to-day. In comparison, social work is handicapped by its brief history, but this does not excuse 'the lack of interest of many workers in the social services, and even among the academics, in evaluating the results of their work . . .' [10]. However, we can claim now that a change is under way; social work is beginning to respond to the healthy if astringent demand to show the value of what it offers, not just in terms of the number of persons served nor by descriptions of what has been done, but by attempts to measure what difference has been brought about and with what side effects.

The Old Age Project in Southwark [21], to which I referred in Chapter I, is the first attempt in this country to test experi-mentally what difference it makes to old people in need of local authority services if one group—randomly chosen—is helped by experienced social workers with training and the other, also random, group is helped by experienced staff who have not had a professional training in social work. The old people were assessed independently by a research social worker and by a physician with psychiatric training, neither knowing which old people were in the experimental group. After some 10 months, the old people who still remained in the community were once again assessed independently and the differences in methods between the two groups of workers analysed and related to differences in outcome; I am glad to be able to report that there were some! No one, least of all those who promoted this project, would expect the results of this first and complex experiment to be definitive or easy to interpret but the results and the method-ology should provide an impetus to further work of this kind.

Tizard among others has pleaded for the experimental study of developments in welfare institutions of various kinds. In one sense we *are* experimenting all the time in the social services, for we are trying out new things, but we are not trying to do so in such a way that we can learn systematically from new experience. Tizard [2] asks for 'an experimental social science which will plan variations in practice in a systematic way in order to study the functioning of social institutions . . . Experiment and evaluation could be a most powerful tool in bringing about social change.' The social services, including the health services, are big business and no commercial industry could develop for long if it spent so small a part of its budget on the attempt to understand what its objectives are, just what it is doing and to what effect. Experiment and evaluation in the social services are of course handicapped by the difficult ethical issues which arise.

5. PROFESSIONAL EDUCATION

Many of these impediments to fruitful co-operation prompt questions about how students are educated for the professions and especially for inter-professional practice. One underlying difficulty is that training for the professions is given by older generations whose experience and pattern of practice will be inapposite for a good deal of the trainees' lives because things change so quickly; and training programmes rarely include the necessity of give and take with other professions.

The Report of the Royal Commission on Medical Education makes it clear that an essential part of the medical student's education is to learn how to treat human beings in trouble and that all students should be taught to recognize the effect of their own behaviour upon other people. It stresses the importance of social aspects of individual patients and adds that, though the community background of the individual case is now recognized to be the concern of every clinical teacher, it is still inadequately provided for in the undergraduate course. It recommends that students should at the start have an historical and comparative introduction to the medical needs of society and the role of the doctor and other health workers. Teaching by sociologists and social administrators, it says, should be specifically adapted to the needs of these students and teaching in the social aspects of medicine should be integrated with the clinical work of the students during the undergraduate course and the intern year. 'The student', says the Report, 'has to be made aware in the hospital ward and in the home, as well as in the classroom, why patients and families behave as they do in situations of illness; of the social and cultural factors which influence the patients' expectations and responses; of the problems for doctor, patient and family in the management of illness and handicap in the community; of the social, ethnic, occupational and psychological forces which can hinder prevention and treatment; and the difficulties of communication, and other problems which arise from established expectations about the way a person in a defined situation will behave, particularly in hospital. There is no single way of achieving this aim.'

Classroom teaching, the Report suggests, can sometimes be provided in common with people training for other professions, for instance, students of social administration. But practice is learnt thro' practice; as Jefferys [22] remarked, by dirtying your hands and not just by beautiful courses in behavioural sciences. Students in all the helping professions must acquire early the habit of *using* the knowledge they gain about what the other professions can provide. This presumes an in-built inter-professional training which, so far as I am aware, no one has yet worked out. This is certainly wanted also outside medicine; 'many social workers', says the Seebohm Report, 'need to learn far more about the doctor's job and what is happening in medicine today'—and this learning should not be confined to the classroom.

This exposure to the practice of parallel disciplines will not be easy to work out; economical methods of learning in this way will call for a good deal of experiment and the investment of resources. But it could be infinitely worthwhile and I shall return to the idea.

The Todd Report emphasized the need for post-graduate medical students, especially in psychiatry, community medicine and general practice, to learn about social studies related to medicine, for instance in the use of the social services, in planning the discharge of patients, in rehabilitation and job placement. But the need patently extends beyond what is normally thought of as post-graduate training. The day is long past in every profession when the student on qualifying could assume that he had packed a bag which, with the occasional replacement, would last a lifetime. Refresher courses should bring professionals up-to-date about changes in related professions, acquaint them with the quiet revolutions as well as the noisy. There should be demonstrations of fresh ways of collaboration, for the habit of teamwork can atrophy. These refresher courses could also provide opportunities for indispensable talk about mutual dissatisfactions: without doubt, there will be ample material! Everyone who speaks on collaboration today is obliged to say that conflict is also necessary but there is seldom difficulty in ensuring conflict—the difficulty is in using it constructively. Let us hope it will be concerned not with empires and status but with what is in the best interest of patients and clients.

It has been suggested that I should include something about the professional preparation of social workers and about the place of the National Institute for Social Work Training. I have acknowledged that shoemakers are convinced there is nothing like leather; they also know that there is no talk like shop talk, so I agreed with alacrity.

Traditionally most social workers in Britain were trained in universities where, as a rule, the strictly professional (I almost said clinical) course normally lasts one year following two or three years' study of society and individual development.[1] Universities are now beginning to offer integrated four year courses in social work and also two year post-graduate professional courses.

Until some ten years ago, fewer than 10 per cent of social workers in local authority health and welfare departments had completed full-time courses designed to prepare them for their jobs. In those days it was necessary to argue at length that social workers, even with mentally disordered people, *ought* to have training for this work. Many influential persons maintained

[1] For many years the Institute of Medical Social Workers also provided a post-graduate course in social work.

that all the social worker required was a good heart, common-
sense and such skill as could be plucked from the hedgerows of
experience. It was against this background that the Younghusband Working Party [24] recommended the urgent extension
of university provision and recommended that courses of training for social work should be established in local authority
Colleges of Further Education. Today, about 30 per cent of
workers in health and welfare departments are professionally
trained or have completed courses in social science and administration and the proportion is growing. This is a remarkable
achievement, but the gap still to be filled before the community
can be sure of receiving a proper professional service is very
large indeed. Social work courses in Colleges of Further
Education normally consist of two years' combined social study
and professional training. All professional courses include a
substantial proportion of field practice under careful supervision
and a major obstacle to the more rapid expansion of training has
been the profession's proper insistence on the provision of field
teaching and supervision at a sufficiently high level.

The professional courses are still nearly all in social casework
but in some an introduction is provided also to community
work and residential care. Since the publication of the Williams
Report [24] on the staffing of residential accommodation, there
has been an extension to other forms of residential care of the
kind of staff training which until then was virtually confined to
the child care field. There has also been a new emphasis on
the common elements in all kinds of residential work; at
the same time there is a clearer appreciation of the distinc-
tion between residential care which is mainly concerned with
providing a substitute home and that where the primary aim
is therapy.

Over the last twelve years or so there has been a revolution in
the quantity and quality of training and this owes much to the
work of Eileen Younghusband. It was the Report which bears
her name that urged that a staff college should be established
to do for social work what similar institutions are doing, for
instance, in administration and defence. As a result of this
recommendation the National Institute for Social Work Training came into being. The National Institute claims no mono-

poly; all its activities are the concern also of other educational institutions and professional bodies; the Institute does, however, claim that it brings these activities together in a way which enhances the usefulness of each. It was established in 1961 by the Nuffield Foundation and the Joseph Rowntree Memorial Trust with premises and income guaranteed in the first place for ten years. The backing of these Trusts—and subsequent support from other Foundations—has ensured a degree of independence, the chance to experiment, the opportunity to respond quickly, the feeling that one didn't always have to play safe. For a body of this kind, a degree of 'irresponsibility' is indispensable and it helps to attract a staff of exceptional calibre, in a fiercely competitive world. The dictionary says, not very helpfully, that a staff college is a college that trains staff officers. As I understand it, and in this context, a staff college should pursue two related aims. In the first place, it should provide the opportunity for trained and experienced workers who occupy—or are expected to occupy—positions of real responsibility to come back to an educational institution for re-charging and retooling, and this includes a fresh examination of professional aims and practice. It should also try itself to carry out some of the experimental projects and research that push back the boundaries of professional knowledge and skill, including skill in training. With this goes the obligation to keep on asking the basic questions about what training should be aiming at and how far it is achieving it.

The National Institute provides a course designed to help experienced practitioners to become effective teachers of social work. The course *is* concerned with methods of training, but even more with purpose. It also offers courses—some of them of the sandwich variety—to enable senior practitioners to come back for a refresher course in core subjects and to choose one out of several options designed to take them further in some important current development. These courses include substantial supervised field practice.

Short 'refresher' courses on new developments in, for instance, management, social planning, evaluation and community participation, are offered for heads of social work departments in local authorities and voluntary bodies; refresher courses on similar lines are provided for senior social workers and for social work teachers.

One important feature of the work is concerned with what I suppose the Defence Staff College would call 'combined operations'. Social work has been split among the various separate services—child care, mental health, medical social work, etc., and the National Institute has tried to provide a forum for the discussion of common aims, common practice and the common client. We have also attempted combined operations with other professions, residential study conferences arranged with the Society of Medical Officers of Health, with local authority Clerks and Treasurers and with educationalists. Another example of combined operations are meetings to discuss topics where many professions converge, such as environmental studies, the Skeffington Report on People and Planning or the phenomenon known as rootless youth.

We have a research department and I have already referred to some of its work. It is directed to learning how to do research in a field where very little has been done in the country; it is also concerned with how to teach research methods to social workers and administrators. But above all it is concerned with conveying the importance of objective and systematic enquiry in social work, and encouraging all concerned to 'consume' research, to study it critically and with a view to application. It attempts to compensate for the fact that social work has, academically, tended to produce too many angels and too few devils. The specific research projects are, of course, directed to questions that should help in the practice and teaching of social work.

Related to research are experimental projects such as the attachment of a social worker to a group general practice, a new venture in community social work, and an attempt to demonstrate ways of improving training on the job.

The Institute has published over 20 volumes in its eight years of life. A good many of these present research which has proved useful for practice and for policy and which, without editorial help, would have remained mute in the mortuaries of unpublished theses for higher degrees. Of course, we have a library which is directed especially to the needs of advanced students and researchers.

Almost against our first intention, we have found ourselves becoming an international centre. A succession of senior Fulbright Scholars has added riches to our store and researchers from overseas are now a regular and most welcome part of our pattern. A few advanced students are accepted and our staff gain from their own travel abroad to teach and consult.

Speaking from the most prejudiced of positions, I believe that a body like this can probably make a useful contribution in other professions.

6. CONCLUSIONS

In this chapter I have tried to trace the factors that impede the practice of regular teamwork between doctors and workers in the other social services and what can be done to improve collaboration. One influence is the feeling that the services are hard to reach, not reliably there when wanted and, in some areas, not dependable.

Of course, poor communication is by definition an obstacle to collaboration; similarly, organizations and administration— created only to facilitate the purpose of the services, may discourage the fresh look and frustrate easy access to the totality of care.

Professional pride and prejudice may also work against easy and smooth co-operation; the issue of confidentiality may be used to justify a refusal to fraternize with the enemy—for so other professionals may be regarded—except at the price of total surrender. Of course, professional education and re-education can determine attitudes and establish habits.

I have concluded by giving a sketchy outline of the training of social workers and the role of the National Institute for Social Work Training.

REFERENCES

1 CROSSMAN, R. (1969) *Paying for the Social Services*, Fabian Society Pamphlet.
2 TIZARD, J. (1966) *The Integration of the Handicapped in Society*, London: Extext Publications.
3 REVANS, R. (1964) *Standards for Morale: Cause and Effect in Hospitals*, London: Oxford University Press.
4 FORDER, A. *et al.* (1969) 'Communications in the Health Service', *Social and Economic Administration* vol. 3 no. 1.
5 HOOPER, D. (1969) 'Conflict and Co-operation in Hospital Care', *Medical Social Work* June 1969.
6 CENTRAL HEALTH SERVICES COUNCIL (1963) *Communications Between Doctors, Nurses and Patients*, H.M.S.O.
7 — (1961) Standing Maternity and Midwifery Advisory Committee. 'Human relations in obstetrics', H.M.S.O.
8 GODBER, G. (1969) *The Future Place of the Personal Physician*, University of Chicago: Center for Health Administration Studies.
9 DEPARTMENT OF HEALTH AND SOCIAL SECURITY (1970) *The Future Structure of the National Health Service*, H.M.S.O.
10 *Report of the Committee on the Local Authority Personal Social Services* (1968) H.M.S.O. Cmnd. 3703.
11 ROBINSON, K. (1967) *Partnership in Medical Care*, University of Glasgow.
12 *Report of the Mental Deficiency Committee* (1929) H.M.S.O.
13 KUSHLICK, A. *A Method of Evaluating the Effectiveness of a Community Health Service*, New York: U.N. Study Group on Meaning and Implications of Community Care 1969.
14 *Report of the Committee of Enquiry into Allegations at the Ely Hospital, Cardiff* (1969) H.M.S.O. Comnd. 3975.
15 MORRIS, P. (1969) *Put Away*, London: Routledge and Kegan Paul.
16 CARR-SAUNDERS, A. M. and WILSON, P. A. (1933) *The Professions*, London: Oxford University Press.
17 BROTHERSTON, J. H. F. (1969) 'Change and the National Health Service', *Scottish Medical Journal* **14**, 130
18 Report of the General Medical Services Committee of the British Medical Association, *British Medical Journal* 27 Sept. 1969.
19 *Report of the Royal Commission on Medical Education* (1968) H.M.S.O. Comnd. 3569.
20 TITMUSS, R. M. (1968) *Commitment to Welfare*, London: George Allen and Unwin.
21 GOLDBERG, E. M. *et al.* (1970) *Helping the Aged: A Field Experiment in Social Work*, London: George Allen and Unwin, National Institute for Social Work Training Series.
22 JEFFERYS, M. (1969) 'Sociology and Medicine', *Lancet* 17 June 1969.

23   *Report of the Working Party in Social Workers on the Local Authority Health & Welfare Services* (1959) H.M.S.O.

24   COMMITTEE ON THE STAFFING OF RESIDENTIAL HOMES (1967) *Caring for People*, London: George Allen and Unwin, National Institute for Social Work Training Series.

CHAPTER III

I. THE COMMON PROBLEMS

SOMEHOW, the attitudes and the apparatus of a working partnership must be established between medicine and other helping professions. It looks as if little short of revolution will bring this about and revolutions often leave patterns of behaviour, attitudes, and relationships remarkably as they were before. When the dust—and the papers—have settled, things go on much the same; only the names seemed to have changed. Revolutions that aim to produce differences in attitudes and ways of working have to be cultivated over a period; they call for a continuing process of education for all concerned and not only for changes in legislation and organization, necessary as these are. Learning to work together is likely to prove a hard job and with this sobering thought I turn to ask which are the common problems and how can they be identified early.

Hopefully, not every patient or every medical problem requires the intervention of other social services. The sensible use of limited resources depends partly on doctors knowing the sort of case in which workers in other social services can make a significant contribution—and knowing these cases early. In those few general practices that have included a social worker as a member of the team, it appears that the doctors referred under ten per cent of patients to this worker. In the Caversham practice, about two-thirds of patients seen by the social worker were women (partly it is suggested because the family and its problems are traditionally regarded as their business); two-thirds of the patients were single or no longer married and one-third were elderly or old [1]. The distribution by social class coincided very closely with the census distribution in the borough; social work help appears to be needed and accepted no less by patients in social classes one and two than in classes three to five. The problems with which the doctors tended to ask for the social worker's help were complex, with inter-related symptoms and they proved hard to analyse. In the main, these were family problems, concerned with relations between the spouses, parent and child, and the wider family.

The question is not only how to ensure that patients who could benefit from the other social services are enabled to get this help, but how to ensure that the patients referred are the ones most in need and most likely to be helped this way. The question applies also in hospitals where, according to a recent study in the U.S.A. [2] the doctors' selection of cases for the social work department was pretty arbitrary.

My colleague E. M. Goldberg [3] has attempted a working classification of the situations where there is a *prima facie* case for social work help, and I have used—and she may feel misused—her scheme. First there are *families with chronically handicapped members*, as in the earlier illustrations of spina bifida and paraplegia. People who are profoundly deaf from infancy present a complex of problems for all concerned and perhaps especially for the psychiatrist (for how do psychiatrists commuciate with deaf people? [4]), problems for educationalists, psychologists, and the whole range of personal social services and—if only they would see it—for experts in linguistics. These problems are often desperate, and they are still hardly explored. It is true today, as Dame Eileen Younghusband said ten years ago, that the deaf are the blind spot of society's conscience.

Mental illness and mental retardation form a second category. Numerically burdensome and oppressive in other ways are those people whose mental or personality handicap is not consistent or, so to speak, reliable. Like Hamlet they are but mad north–north–west: when the wind is southerly they know a hawk from a handsaw. Here perhaps the lines between health and social problems are most blurred and here the burden must continue to be carried in the first place by the family and the family doctor. This group will overlap with those patients with *persistent stress symptoms*, vague psychosomatic complaints who, in one group practice, amounted to a quarter of the patients referred by the doctors to the social worker. Morris [5] has referred to this psychosomatic group—with its perhaps rising prevalence—as 'the most elusive area of epidemiology'.

Crisis situations are often an indication of the need for other social services: terminal illness, death, the birth of a severely handicapped child, attempted suicide and major accidents that involve changes in role and way of life.

Other indications are related to the *difficult periods in the life cycle* such as old age and the time from adolescence to young manhood when the turbulence of our culture appears to concentrate dramatically. This of course is not peculiar to *our* culture, for did not the shepherd in *The Winter's Tale* say 'I would there were no age between sixteen and three-and-twenty, or that youth would sleep out the rest; for there is nothing in the between but getting wenches with child, wronging the ancientry, stealing, fighting'.

Another category may be the *contemporary or fashionable concerns*; at the moment, examples are drug addiction and the syndrome known—most deplorably—as the 'battered baby'; delinquency is the one contemporary concern that is permanent!

We start with broad categories like these and they can be of great use in alerting the doctor but, of course, it is essential to work out, on the basis of recorded experience and operational studies, more precise criteria for those cases where social work help is indicated. This problem should be tackled at a centre for inter-professional studies where one would also consider how workers in the other social services could be better equipped to recognize the indications of medical need. One example of the contribution that lay workers can make in promoting medical treatment is provided in Sorsby's [6] studies of blindness. The decline in the proportion of blindness in later life is due, of course, to treatment provided through the National Health Service. But Sorsby's studies indicate that referrals to the blind register, very often the first step, are due mainly to lay people and especially to the officers of the Supplementary Benefits Commission. Sorsby's studies left at least this reader wondering whether there may not be much unnecessary blindness suffered without proper social support, among old people who are not visited by officers of the Supplementary Benefits Commission. Medical practitioners, it appeared, had failed to notice, diagnose or do something about remediable blindness and the visiting officers of the Supplementary Benefits Commission were acting as a long stop.

2. THE QUESTION OF REFERRAL

So far I have tried to show some of the common problems and suggested the need for serviceable criteria for recognizing those cases which should be referred by doctors to the social services and by workers in these services to doctors. But is 'referral' the right word? One experienced community physician was visibly nettled by the term and said that a doctor should never 'refer' because referral can so easily be a way of rejecting a patient, a method of dumping the troublesome or even tedious case. 'Never refer,' said this doctor, 'share cases instead.' Referral can also take the form of telling people in other professions just what they should do; Moon [7] quotes examples of quite specific instructions by consultants to social workers for after-care rather than requests for social assessment and for after-care within this context.

Even when doctors wish not to refer but 'share' a case, it is easy for the patient to get the impression that somehow he is being shunted off. The patient must know that this is not a dismissal by the doctor of the physical problem, that social work is not forced upon him but offered as an appropriate part of the total service needed for this case. This sense of genuine partnership within the hospital or practice cannot be conveyed unless it is genuinely there; here is another problem for a centre for inter-professional studies, and I shall want to return to that later.

3. SEEBOHM AND THE COMMUNITY PHYSICIAN

Bertrand Russell is reported to have said that if the child about to be weaned could speak, he would look up from the breast and protest 'Surely you can't expect me to change the habits of a lifetime at my age!' Proposals for major changes in organization can never be universally welcome and a previous Heath Clark Lecturer, Karl Evang [8] has contrasted the medical professions' willingness to accept and use the findings of science with its reluctance to acknowledge that new conditions make new settings imperative.

We meet at a time when big changes are clearly imminent. The development of unified district health services is forecast, outside local government but eventually with co-terminous boundaries and in some ways closer links with the community than hitherto.

It is now taken for granted that responsibility for community health must be part of an integral health service. Public health developed in Britain in the middle decades of the nineteenth century to meet a situation which to a large extent public health itself has transformed, not merely by the specific measures it has carried through but by brilliant, courageous and inspired leadership which merits a series of war histories to itself. But what served yesterday may not be right for tomorrow; different design of services, personnel and 'philosophy' may be necessary, including different relations with other professions. One of the weaknesses of our public services—perhaps all services—is their reluctance to ask, hard enough and often enough, whether their organization, objectives and even their personnel are really meeting the demands of changing situations.

This point is brought out sharply in Reports issued by the Queen's Institute of District Nursing [9] which demonstrate that our present organization does not promote co-operation even between nurses in public health departments and doctors in hospitals or in general practice. This is in every sense the burden of these documents, one of which finds little evidence of rational distribution of care between hospital and community services, and a misunderstanding of roles and failures in communication. In the six hospitals covered by the enquiry, in nearly 80 per cent of the cases there was no indication of *any* request for community services. The other report *Feeling the Pulse* [10] says that 'Communication with general practice is seen to be minimal' and 'There was surprisingly little personal contact between the doctors and nurses . . . One nurse, who had been in her area more than a year, had never met any of her patients' doctors'. It has been pointed out that these two Reports may fail to give credit to those places where things have improved, such as local authorities where nursing staff work closely with general practice; those where early discharge schemes in midwifery or surgery are well developed and areas where local co-ordination have provided a basis for the Best Buy concept for hospital development.

Proposals for changing the organization and responsibilities of the local authority personal social services—and incidentally improving their relations with the medical profession—are set out in the Seebohm Report; and legislation to implement some of these proposals is now before Parliament.

It is sad though not exceptional that so little discussion, either criticism or support, of this Report has come from any except the professions that have most at stake. The same of course goes for education, law and the civil service; it is teachers, lawyers, and civil servants who ardently debate changes in these services always, of course, on the grounds that they are concerned with the public interest. But historically proposals for change always clash head-on with professional resistance if they involve yielding one iota of power or accepting as colleagues any who might challenge a monopoly of skill.

The Seebohm proposals bring together in one local authority department—still quite a small department in staff and spending—all those personal social services that are designed to meet needs that are not primarily medical. Of course, there will be medical aspects of the problems dealt with, and of course these must be treated by *medical services*; this is not in dispute. The issue is about other services such as guidance about the range of provision available for frail old people, social support for mentally disordered men and women and their families, help with personal and social difficulties, the provision of residential accommodation that is both comfortable and alive, and winning local acceptance and interest for these Homes. Does work like this call primarily for a doctor's skill either in doing it or in directing it? More important, can it be that the work calls for knowledge, skill and experience different from those the doctor acquires during his training and practice?

A recent leading article in The Medical Officer [11] argued that the guiding rule should be that all things medical must remain in medical hands and conceded 'that all things sociological (their term, not mine) might well go to our social work colleagues'. Indeed, the writer of this article went further, asking does it have to be the M.O.H. who decides that granny can no longer look after herself, remembering that granny has a G.P.? Does it have to be the M.O.H. who is consulted when some parents decide they are not going to accept their new-born mongol child, again remembering that other medical men are involved?

The positive case for Seebohm is first that it proposes a coherent organization, one that will be easy for clients and other professions to know, to use—and hold accountable. With one organization responsible, it will be easier to distribute resources according to the needs of the public and easier to undertake comprehensive planning, including preventive work.

But Seebohm also promotes what some commentators have called 'a new philosophy', advocating that, like the National Health Service, the personal social services should become a citizen's service, community based, family oriented, available to all and good enough for all to want to use. 'This new department', says the Report, 'will, we believe, reach far beyond the discovery and rescue of social casualties; it will enable the greatest possible number of individuals to act reciprocally, giving and receiving service for the well-being of the whole community.'

The Report stresses how essential it is that the new department should work closely with the medical services and especially with community medicine. 'The needs of the local population should . . . be diagnosed and policy should be decided, plans formulated and carried out jointly, and with full consideration of the mutual consequences for all the various services.' The Report is optimistic—and bold—enough to argue that by recognizing and accepting these differences in function and responsibilities, a far *more* fertile co-operation could be achieved than exists today, one that would make more use, and much more appropriate use, of the doctor's contribution. This is partly what Seebohm is about and the Report urges that 'Together (doctors and social workers) might be more effective in diagnosis as well as in providing care and support for the many in serious social and emotional difficulties who cannot at present be offered it'.

The new social service departments will depend heavily on the help of family doctors, community physicians and clinical consultants in diagnosing local needs, planning the services and appraising them; in advising on admissions to and the running of residential homes, half-way houses, hostels, clubs and day care establishments, including nurseries; in providing services for various special groups and individuals; in public education and community relations, and for staff training.

Morris [5] has said that responsibility for achieving the closest co-ordination among the clinical and social services will be 'the first task of the community physician of tomorrow'. I would add that it must be among the first responsibilities of the director of the new social service department.

4. GENERAL PRACTICE

This is a difficult moment to speculate on the brave new patterns of collaboration that may emerge, partly because it is still not easy to think of national health provisions except as separated services. Hopefully, there will soon be a unification of the health services and that in itself should make partnership with other social services easier, but there is no assurance that this *will* happen. It is possible, as some Jeremiahs have prophesied, that the setting up of an integrated health service outside local government and an integrated social service department within the local authority will make divisions deeper, collaboration more difficult and partnership just a bad joke. Whatever new structure is established, some resentment will be only human among those who in consequence suffer in status or responsibility.

It is vital that these new organizations for health and social service should get off to a flying start and that patients and clients should not suffer in the transition. This shows up the need, when Bills and Papers, green or white, are published, to set up some machinery to look at mutual consequences, to anticipate snags, to study how to build-in ways of working together from the start. This would, of course, be just the job for a centre for inter-professional studies if only we had one. Meanwhile it must not go by default.

Godber [12], looking to the future of medical provision in this country, has forecast 'a complex, at the centre of which is the hospital as the main support of practice centres dispersed through the community. In this way general practice is supported by the specialities, and the service the community requires in any area of medicine is partly provided by each'.

Single-handed general practice is now said to be on the way out; the G.P. is becoming a team man and in a few years the normal pattern will be the group of family doctors working in association with nurses, midwives, and part-time social workers by some arrangement with the local authority social service department.

Thought has gone a long way beyond the health centres as they were proposed originally. Brotherston [13], for instance, writing about the health centre at Stranraer, has said that a health centre by itself does not necessarily change the quality or satisfaction of the doctor's work, although its facilities may make work easier; group practice does not necessarily enhance the standard of medicine, although it may lighten the doctor's job. The essential spark necessary to warm general practice into new life, he says, lies in the professional stimulus and interaction.

Since Seebohm, the term 'health and social service centre' has come into use and in a few places into partial practice. It is to be hoped that there will be a variety of experiments, including centres for health services and the area teams proposed in the new social service departments. All these experiments should be monitored and evaluated. We ought also to learn from other countries, including attempts in the U.S.A. [14] to establish what has been called 'a prototype for a new form of human service organization charged with responsibilities which engage traditional health and welfare services'. Put like that it sounds grand enough for anything!

Over the past decade, important innovations have taken place in general practice in working with other professions: health visitors and home nurses, 'practice nurses' and, in several pioneer projects, social workers [15].

The work in the Caversham Centre confirms that a group family practice is an excellent pickup point for people in great need of the help that social work and other social services can provide, the great majority of whom had never been in touch with any social service agency. It has also shown again that medical symptoms can be a respectable way of presenting social problems; by contrast it may look like a confession of personal failure if you have to admit you have come about your difficult relationships or your incompetence in managing your other affairs and besides, you may not know it. The need has been demonstrated for an easy and natural way of sharing cases that come, perhaps without admitting or even being aware of it, for something other than help with their 'health'. For some patients, the social worker may be an enabler, acting partly as an interpreter in contacts between doctors, voluntary and statutory social services and their patients, sometimes promoting flexibility in services so as to meet the types of social need which patients bring to their practitioners. Incidentally, the research social worker in this project has suggested that patients might be included in discussions about their own medical-social treatment much more than they are in general at present. Patients, after all, do not 'belong' to their doctors, or clients to their social workers; they are not disposable property.

We have all been taught that it is wrong to generalize from one example and we are all tempted when we have two. In the Caversham project and in experiments reported by Forman and Fairbairn [16] and others, the doctors and the social workers worked together smoothly and effectively in a partnership that developed as they gained experience of each other. Forman dismisses the idea that the social worker may be a threat to the doctor-patient relationship, provided there is mutual confidence and a high standard of communication between general practitioner and social worker. He adds 'As the experiment proceeded there was perhaps some shift away from asking the (social worker) to perform some specific function in a case, towards bringing her into a problem for her specialist knowledge and skills, and expecting her to proceed in any way she found indicated'. Another worker has stressed the importance of staff making time to talk with one another and the need for social workers to develop flexible methods of working, including hours that match the doctors', in order to go along with the requirements of the practice.

After these mutually cordial compliments of family doctors and social workers who have worked together, it has been suggested that this pattern should spread quickly, aiming even at one social worker for each group general practice. The recent Report of the Scottish Working Party [17] under the chairmanship of W. J. M. MacKenzie quotes proposals for one whole-time social worker to 10 000 patients and argues that this figure is unrealistic as an immediate target. In my view, it is doubtful whether there will ever be enough social workers for this sort of provision and it is questionable whether this is in general the most effective or economical way of using them. More recorded experiments are needed, and one is now being promoted by the Camden Public Health Department, on how the 'laboratory' type of projects we have known in group practices can be applied more generally, for instance by finding out how one social worker can work with two or more practices. Incidentally, attachment to a health centre or a group practice should not for any of the workers concerned mean detachment from their own professional grouping; membership and not attachment is the right relationship to a group.

5. HOSPITALS, CONSULTANTS AND THE SOCIAL SERVICES

At present nearly 90 per cent of medical social workers work within the walls of hospitals and only about 10 per cent in local authority or other services. Medical social workers constitute one of the most highly trained groups of social workers; they and psychiatric social workers are specially prepared in their training to work with doctors in the treatment of illness. Medical social workers are hospital-based for historical reasons which go back in part to the poverty of so many sick people, hence the old name of almoners, first applied in the Royal Free Hospital, and an origin to be proud of. These historical reasons no longer prevail and medical social workers themselves have been asking (as the psychiatric social workers asked earlier) is this the best way to provide social work services for sick people in the last decades of the twentieth century? Should it survive in the new set-up proposed by Seebohm? Is a hospital social work service—

whether the hospital be general or psychiatric—able to provide
continuity of care from early recognition by the family doctor,
through the preparation for hospital and the treatment there,
on to discharge and back to the care of the general practitioner
and the social support and rehabilitation that may be needed?
The plans for rehabilitation, physical or psychiatric, may need
to start even before the patient is admitted to hospital. It is
doubtful if medical social workers, based mainly in hospitals,
can achieve this continuity of care. Even in a hospital with a
long and fine tradition of co-operation and a distinguished social
work department, fewer than a quarter of the referrals came
from doctors [18]. Other studies show that referrals for social
assessment or direct social casework were rare; a high proportion were requests to carry out quite specific jobs and the social
workers said that sometimes they wondered if they were serving
as disposal officers.

It would, of course, be important to ensure that hospitals
would not be worse off in the social services available to them if
they were served by the new local authority department, even
though these services were differently organized.

The service might well be better, for it could not then occur,
as it occurs often now, that hospitals—and particularly mental
hospitals—find themselves altogether without social workers,
because one or two have left. Secondment of social workers to
work with hospitals, involving special long term association, is
perfectly feasible, as experience has shown. The *patients* most
in need should be better off through earlier recognition
and continuity of care before hospital, through hospital, and
after.

Health service in the community must of course include
teamwork between hospital and family doctors; it has been said
'They need to understand each other's jobs, to share information and to agree on the individual programme, as so often is
not the case today', and the examples quoted earlier, from the
rare spina bifida to common old age suggests this *medical* teamwork is often not happening, that hospital doctors tend not to
have adequate working contacts with general practitioners or
with the local health authority—the patients suffer and a valu-
able opportunity is lost in the training of junior doctors in

co-operation between hospital and general practice. The point I am making here chimes in with the recommendation of the Cogwheel Report [19] that within the hospital there should be a group of clinicians to take an active part in the co-ordination and planning of services and provide effective liaison with the community services outside the hospital.

Soon, we hope, it will no longer be possible to think of separate Ten Year (or other) Plans for hospitals and other social services. The need for hospitals is so patently influenced by what alternative provision is available in the community when admission is considered and again when discharge seems appropriate. A co-ordinated policy is required to which all hospitals (in-patient and out-patient, day, night, short stay, long stay, peripatetic and open hospitals), general practitioners, community medicine and all the other social services make their appropriate and necessarily changing contribution. This is where the concept of the Best Buy hospital comes in; the idea, which the name fails to convey, is to provide a district service in which a particular kind of hospital is only one constituent and it is planned as it is mainly because of what is expected to be done outside.

6. A CENTRE FOR INTER-PROFESSIONAL STUDIES

In no profession today is the patient or client with a serious problem likely to be the responsibility of one specialist alone. Teamwork is imperative both within professions (and this does not happen so easily or so effectively as we sometimes presume) and between professions. The question is, how to ensure that if a case requires it—and the case may be an individual patient, a family or a whole community—there will be a total team approach. And the answer to this question is direct and brief: no one knows. The one thing we can be sure of is that a team approach is far too complex for it just to happen. As the Seebohm Report says, 'It is idle to think that such new patterns of medical social team work required by newly recognized medical social needs can easily be established'. And Butterfield [20] wrote of the Thamesmead experiment that it was 'quickly apparent why integrated medical care and welfare does not just happen: it requires the arduous pursuit of ideas and a great deal of effort and sometimes tact in communicating them to the interested parties'.

So far, the clamour (to which I have added my share) has been for more goodwill, more understanding of needs and opportunities, more listening to one another and more training about other services and how to use them. One experienced community physician has criticized the Seebohm approach because, he argues, it has not faced the realities of inter-professional team-work, that it is naïvely optimistic about what can be attained by independent voluntary co-operation between— or even within—professions by such conventional means as referring patients, case conferences, sermons on collaboration or even secondment to work together. He asked, in effect, is it better to start at the beginning by looking into the possibilities of inter-disciplinary and inter-professional training or must we try later to build bridges over moraines of mutual ignorance, misunderstanding and ingrained suspicion.

There are, of course, inherent difficulties in the way of any attempt to achieve a fresh approach to the problems of team-work, not least the sheer pressure on the doctor's time when he is a student and later in practice. Everyone concerned with medical education calls for more time for the particular part of the syllabus they are interested in and the same goes for so-called refresher courses for keeping the experienced professional workers up-to-date with new developments. It is also a complication that there can be no uniform pattern of team-work; what works well in one setting, such as a general hospital, may not serve in community medicine.

And yet, in spite of difficulties, we are in a sense committed; we cannot escape the attempt and I hope we do not want to. Since the Report of the Royal Commission on Mental Health with its splendid advocacy of community care, we should have learnt that it is not enough to will the end unless we are also ready to contrive the means and the means are not confined to additional resources that money will buy; they include also new ways of working which imply new learning. It will not serve to change the structure unless we are also prepared to provide the training that can make the new structure work and this includes some retraining for the established practitioners on whom each profession must depend for a long time ahead.

Against this background, the need becomes clear for a focus for inter-professional studies, a centre to look at difficulties that arise in partnership between professions and to work out ways of promoting this partnership. The particular professions involved must vary according to the nature of the problem. Today, in differing circumstances, they could include medicine, nursing, social work, law, education, economics (for instance for cost benefit analysis), epidemiology (social as well as medical), planning and management. Without doubt, the centre would have to study partnership *within* professions as well as between them; it is essential that the patient or client also should be accepted as one of the partners.

One of the depressing themes throughout these lectures has been failure in collaboration but, as I have mentioned more than once, there are examples of highly successful teamwork and much could be learnt even from the failures, if only we knew how to benefit from the lessons. New models for effective team-work could be set up, designed to explore techniques in a variety of working situations.

This centre should become a place to which field agencies, for instance, hospitals, health centres, social work departments, bring their team-work problems, and this is important for, as McKeown [21] said 'The research worker can't solve all the problems he sees but he's very unlikely to solve those he never sees'. In other words, experienced researchers should be working at the points where appropriate problems for study can be recognized early. This centre would be a laboratory—but not only a laboratory, for it would have responsibility for providing the bridge, still badly needed in the social sciences, between research and the useful application of research findings in the field. The centre should also develop a do-it-yourself methodo-logy for monitoring local field projects so that they may evaluate what they are doing more readily and more objectively.

The centre should be a place where practitioners, teachers and researchers from different fields come together to think and argue, stimulating and challenging each other. This is needed for instance in connection with what has been called 'the spectre' of leadership within a team. When the team is small and develops likemindedness, the role of leader may move—almost without noticing—from member to member, according to the salient problem at any given time. In the larger, heterogeneous team, especially if decisions are grave and urgent, there is a greater danger of compromise and indecision. The centre could help to develop 'the devices of leadership' that will give effect to interdependent team work.

The first aim of the Centre must be to know more about the nature of teamwork, the characteristics of effective partnership and the factors that impede it. It must also aim to *communicate* all this and in doing so must work together with the professional schools, taking advantage of the great fillip provided in the Todd Report. How can good foundations for collaboration be laid at the preclinical stage (or whatever is the appropriate term in other professions) as well as at the clinical stage, in classrooms and in the work places, where perforce partnership must be learnt in practice. This exposure to parallel disciplines in practice will not be easy to work out; economical methods of learning in this way (and they *must* be economical especially in time) will call for a good deal of experiment and a considerable investment of resources.

The Todd Report recommends that accommodation for teaching should be shared with students in fields related to medicine and it points out that health centres and group practice should provide practical examples for learning teamwork between doctors and related social services; there are also examples in public health departments. The place of learning *is* important but the core of the learner's preparation for professional practice is his relation with his teachers. If it was necessary to ask where are the teachers of community medicine [22], it is even more necessary to ask, where are the teachers of inter-professional knowledge and practice, and the answer is likely to prove even more baffling. Teaching the teachers will be a central task.

It is vital that new thinking and new ways of inter-professional practice should reach those established workers who carry responsibility in the field today and tomorrow, and for this a range of devices will be needed including demonstration centres, short courses, publications and small conferences. The Cog-wheel Report, it may be remembered, proposed a series of short conferences for the whole profession as part of a multi-disciplin-ary approach to the problems it was considering. In-service training, as Caplan [23] wrote 'demands a major expenditure of time and effort, rather than constituting a luxury to be allotted minor consideration as an embellishment . . .' It is comforting to realize that in these activities, everyone will be a teacher and everyone a student.

I believe that this idea of an inter-professional centre is worth kicking about and dare I hope that some Foundation may be ready to join in the kicking.

7. CONCLUSION

If things went the way they should many an occasion of this kind would end with a vote of thanks from the speaker to those benefactors who have obliged him to read more widely, think harder and argue more vigorously about his subject than he has done hitherto. May I, therefore, start a precedent and move my own heart-felt vote of thanks to the memory of Heath Clark, to those in the University of London who were responsible for the remarkable invitation that reached me, to friends in the London School of Hygiene, the National Institute for Social Work training and elsewhere who have helped me, and who have been forbearing even when I did not follow the guidance I had asked for, and to my generous audience for their encour-agement and fortitude.

REFERENCES

1 GOLDBERG, E. M. *et al.* (1968) 'Social Work in General Practice', *Lancet* 7 September 1968.
2 GORDON, B. and REHR, H. (1969) 'Selectivity Biases in Delivery of Hospital Social Services', University of Chicago Press, *Social Service Review* no. 1, 1969.
3 GOLDBERG, E. M. (1967) 'Early Diagnosis of Social Breakdown', *The Medical World* August 1967.
4 DENMARK, J. C. and RAYMOND W. ELDRIDGE 'Psychiatric Services for the Deaf', *Lancet* 2 August 1969, p. 259.

5 Morris, J. N. (1969) 'Tomorrow's Community Physician', *Lancet* 18 October 1969.

6 Sorsby, A. (1966) *The Incidence and Causes of Blindness in England and Wales*, 1948–62, H.M.S.O. Reports on Public Health and Medical Subjects no. 114.

7 Moon, M. (1964) *The First Two Years. A Study of Some Newly Qualified Medical Social Workers*, London: The Institute of Medical Social Workers.

8 Evang, K. (1960) *Health Service, Society and Medicine*, London: Oxford University Press.

9 Queen's Institute of District Nursing (1968) *Care in the Balance. A Study of Collaboration between Hospital and Community Services.*

10 — (1966) *Feeling the Pulse. A Survey of District Nursing in Six Areas.*

11 *The Medical Officer* (1969) 'Render unto Caesar', 15 August 1969, p. 99.

12 Godber, G. (1969) *The Future Place of the Personal Physician*, University of Chicago: Center for Health Administration Studies.

13 Brotherston, J. H. F. (1969) 'Change and the National Health Service', *Scottish Medical Journal* **14**, 130.

14 Task Force on Social Services (1968) *Services for People*, U.S. Department of Health Education and Welfare.

15 Abel, R. A. (1969) *Nursing Attachments to General Practice*, H.M.S.O. Department of Health and Social Security. Social Science Research Unit Study no. 1.

16 Foreman, J. A. S. and Fairbairn, E. M. (1968) *Social Casework in General Practice*, London: Oxford University Press.

17 Report of a Working Party (1969) *Social Work in Scotland* University of Edinburgh Press.

18 Butrym, Z. (1968) *Medical Social Work in Action*, Occasional Papers in Social and Economic Administration, 26, London: Bell.

19 *First Report of the Joint Working Party on the Organisation of Medical Work in Hospitals* (1967).

20 Butterfield, W. J. H. (1968) *Priorities in Medicine*, London: Nuffield Provincial Hospital Trust.

21 McKeown, T. (1965) *Medicine in Modern Society*, London: Allen & Unwin.

22 Morris, J. N. and Warren, M. D. (1969) 'Where are the Teachers of Community Medicine?', *Lancet* 1 February 1969.

23 Caplan, G. (1961) *An Approach to Community Mental Health*, London: Tavistock Publications.